D
LESS,
LIVE
MORE.

DRINK LESS, LIVE MORE

An Hachette UK Company
www.hachette.co.uk

Vie Books, an imprint of Summersdale Publishers Ltd
Part of Octopus Publishing Group Limited
Carmelite House
50 Victoria Embankment
LONDON
EC4Y 0DZ
UK

www.summersdale.com

Printed and bound in Malta

ISBN: 978-1-78783-032-5

Substantial discounts on bulk quantities of Summersdale books are available to corporations, professional associations and other organizations. For details contact general enquiries: telephone: +44 (0) 1243 771107 or email: enquiries@summersdale.com.

DRINK LESS, LESS, LIVE MORE.

Why Booze Is Not Your Buddy
and How to Cut Down

KATHERINE KAY

Contents

DISCLAIMER

The author and the publisher cannot accept responsibility for any misuse or misunderstanding of any information contained herein, or any loss, damage or injury, be it health, financial or otherwise, suffered by any individual or group acting upon or relying on information contained herein. None of the views or suggestions in this book is intended to replace medical opinion from a doctor who is familiar with your particular circumstances. If you have concerns about your health, please seek professional advice.

IF ONE
OVERSTEPS
THE BOUNDS OF
MODERATION,
THE GREATEST
PLEASURES
CEASE TO
PLEASE.

EPICTETUS

Introduction

When you think about the relationships you have with the people in your life, you may be fully aware that your best friend cracks you up, your boss winds you up, and your family picks you up. But have you stopped to consider the other relationships you have? More specifically, the relationship you have with alcohol? As you've begun reading this book, it's likely you have. And to hazard a guess, maybe you're not entirely happy with how alcohol has been treating you of late – or how you've been treating it. Maybe things are starting to turn toxic. Perhaps the lows are outweighing the highs. Maybe the day-after dread is taking its toll. Your bank balance might be taking a beating. Or you're sick of losing half (or all) of every Sunday marinating in bed.

Stop! There *is* an alternative to drinking to excess. Wait... what? In our booze-soaked society – where "wine o'clock" and those searching for "gin-spiration" are celebrated – perhaps it may not seem so, but it's true. It *is* possible to moderate your alcohol consumption without it ruining your social life. One glass doesn't have to turn into a bottle, one pint need not end with a greasy burger at 3 a.m., and you could even swap your cocktail for a – *gasp* – mocktail. If you're looking to cut down, or stop drinking altogether, this book will help you on your way, offering advice, tips and suggestions on how to think before you drink.

Because life is too short to waste on hangovers.

Facts and Figures

Before we look at what alcohol does to us as individuals, here are some statistics about the scale of alcohol's influence:

- Around 2.3 billion people around the world drink alcohol.
- The highest levels of alcohol consumption are in Europe.
- Alcohol is consumed by more than half the population in America and Europe.
- On average, a person in the world aged 15 or older drinks 6.2 litres (11 pints) of pure alcohol every year.
- Worldwide, 44.8 per cent of alcohol consumed is in the form of spirits, followed by beer at 34.3 per cent, then wine at 11.7 per cent.
- The use and abuse of alcohol results in 3.3 million deaths each year.
- In 2016, there were 11 million deaths globally – alcohol caused an estimated 0.4 million of them.
- Over 200 health conditions are linked to the harmful use of alcohol – including cancers, liver diseases, cardiovascular illnesses and sexually transmitted diseases (due to people having

unprotected sex). This figure also takes into account suicides, alcohol-related violence and road injuries.

- In 2016, around 370,000 alcohol-related deaths were due to road injuries, 150,000 as a result of self-harm, and 90,000 due to violence.
- An estimated 237 million men and 46 million women globally have alcohol-abuse problems.
- In 2016, 57 per cent (3.1 billion people) of the global population aged 15 and over had abstained from drinking alcohol in the previous 12 months.
- When it comes to not drinking alcohol, women abstain for life more often than men (in Britain, 25 per cent of women are teetotal, compared to 18 per cent of men).
- Globally, about 16 per cent of drinkers aged 15 or older partake in "heavy episodic drinking", also known as binge drinking.
- The prevalence of binge drinking has decreased globally from 22.6 per cent in 2000 to 18.2 per cent in 2016.
- In the UK, those aged 16–24 are the least likely to drink of any other age group, with as many as 27 per cent being teetotal, compared to just over a fifth of the broader adult population.

DRINKING STEALS HAPPINESS FROM TOMORROW.

ANONYMOUS

Why Booze Is Not Your Buddy

Alcohol may give you confidence, a feeling of euphoria and the ability to laugh at jokes that aren't funny, but these favourable outcomes are short-lived – the pleasure before the pain. You see, alcohol can impact your life in so many negative ways – with effects on your physical and mental health, relationships, bank balance, appearance, sleep, fertility, sex life, brain function, even your eyesight – that you may find it's not worth drinking it much or at all. Like a toxic friend who drains you of your self-esteem, or a family member who only gets in touch when they need to borrow money, booze can sap your get-up-and-go. It may be a slow process and you may be unaware of it happening, but if you consistently drink heavily over a number of years, it will *catch up with you. Read on to discover how alcohol can impact you and whether it's a "frenemy" you could live without.*

Alcohol Plays Havoc with Your Health

Booze can cause problems galore with your body and mind – both in the short and long term. Here's how:

SHORT-TERM EFFECTS

- Anxiety
- Blackouts
- Diarrhoea
- Disturbed sleep
- Impaired judgement, which can result in injuries or accidents
- Memory loss
- Shaking
- Skin conditions
- Stomach problems
- Stress
- Sweating
- Vomiting
- Weight gain

LONG-TERM EFFECTS

- Brain damage
- Cancer
- Dementia
- Depression
- Heart disease
- High blood pressure
- Liver disease
- Mental-health problems
- Osteoporosis
- Pancreatitis
- Reproductive problems
- Stomach ulcers
- Stroke

Your Mental Health Is Affected

Drinking alcohol affects the neurotransmitters in our brains, which can influence our thoughts, feelings and actions. Alcohol is a depressant, so anxiety, depression and stress can all be amplified by drinking too much. Dehydration, which occurs after drinking alcohol, is also known to cause anxiety. On one end of the scale, you may get "beer fear" – or "hangxiety" – after a night out ("Oh no, please tell me I didn't say/do/dance on that"). At the more serious end of the scale, alcohol is often linked to self-harm and even suicide: alcoholics are up to 120 times more likely to commit suicide than those who are not dependent. If you drink heavily on a regular basis, your brain's levels of serotonin – a chemical that helps to balance your mood – will be lowered, which may lead you to feeling blue and angst-ridden.

Alcohol Causes Cancer

Whether someone binge drinks or spreads their boozing out, cancer doesn't discriminate. Alcohol increases the risk of seven cancers: mouth, upper throat, oesophageal, laryngeal, breast, bowel and liver. And it doesn't have to be excessive amounts of alcohol: the risk of cancer increases even at low levels. Alcohol causes nearly 12,000 cases of cancer a year in the UK, including 8 per cent of cases of breast cancer, the most common form. When we drink, alcohol gets into our bloodstream and harms us in three main ways:

- **Acetaldehyde –** Alcohol is metabolized into a chemical called acetaldehyde, which causes cancer by damaging DNA and preventing cells from repairing this damage.
- **Increased absorption –** Alcohol affects the cells between the throat and mouth, which can make it easier for other carcinogens to be absorbed into the body.
- **Hormone changes –** Some naturally occurring hormones, such as insulin and oestrogen, can increase with the intake of alcohol. High levels of these hormones can cause cancer cells to grow and multiply.

Your Skin Will Suffer

Whenever you drink alcohol, your body becomes dehydrated, which has a massive impact on your skin. It's stripped of the vital nutrients and vitamins it needs to remain healthy, so can become dull and grey. Fortunately, skin reacts quickly to change, so it can return to its usual glowing glory after only a couple of days of cutting back on alcohol. However, over time, heavy drinking can have long-lasting, detrimental effects on your skin. Rosacea, a skin disorder that starts with a propensity to blush profusely and can lead to permanent redness in the face, has been linked to alcohol. Research found that those who drank alcohol had an increased risk of rosacea compared to those who didn't drink, and that this risk increased the more they drank.

Temporary redness in the face is also common when drinking. Alcohol widens blood vessels, causing the face to flush. Usually, your natural colour will return a few hours after drinking; but if you consistently consume too much alcohol, permanent red, spidery veins can appear on your face. When it comes to the skin, alcohol speeds up the ageing process, so if you're a regular drinker, you're more likely to become wrinkly before your time. Booze also decreases the liver's natural level of vitamin A, which is important in maintaining firm and youthful skin by promoting cell turnover and protection from pollution. Dehydration means your skin is dry from the inside out, which makes it wrinkle more quickly and increases the chance of cell damage. Fine lines and creases will appear, and will grow deeper over time.

Spot breakouts and acne can also be caused by alcohol. As it's jam-packed with sugar, alcohol may cause inflammation, which often leads to skin irritation and pimples. Booze can also mess with the balance of hormones and, as our angsty teenage selves may remember, hormones and acne go hand in hand.

Weight Gain Is Likely

Alcohol can make you put on weight – and not just because a large glass of wine contains about the same number of calories as an ice cream, while a pint of cider is as calorific as a sugar-covered doughnut. Yes, the average wine drinker puts on 3 kilograms (7 pounds) of fat a year, but it may not be entirely from the booze itself... Research has shown that drinking alcohol makes you crave food because the neurons in your brain that instigate hunger are activated by alcohol. That's why, come 2 a.m., you may find yourself either raiding your fridge or seeking out late-night fast food. And just as the calories from alcohol are "empty calories" – they have no nutritional value – the junk food you consume as a result of drinking contains very little in the way of nutrients.

Blood Pressure Can Increase

If you have high blood pressure, it means that your heart has to pump harder and your arteries have to carry blood that's flowing under greater pressure. This puts a strain on your heart and arteries, which increases the risk of a stroke or heart attack. High blood pressure (hypertension) can also contribute to vision loss, kidney disease and dementia. Research has shown that about 16 per cent of blood-pressure problems in the US are linked to excessive alcohol consumption. The amount of lipids (fats) present in the bloodstream after drinking alcohol can damage the arteries, causing them to harden, which increases blood pressure and the risk of dangerous clots. Alcohol is also high in calories and sugar, which causes weight gain – a risk factor for high blood pressure. And booze can interfere with the effectiveness of some blood-pressure medications, as well as increasing their negative side effects.

Your Immune System Becomes Weakened

Too much alcohol can interfere with your immune system, meaning you're more vulnerable to illness and infection. If you drink most days, you may notice that you catch coughs, colds, the flu and other illnesses more frequently than those who don't drink. There are three important cells in our immune systems – macrophages, T-cells and B-cells – and drinking to excess reduces the number and function of each. Macrophages are white blood cells that consume anything in our bodies that's not supposed to be there, including cancerous cells. They are the first line of defence against disease. T-cells are antibodies to specific pathogens (bacteria, viruses or other harmful microorganisms). They are the reason vaccines work. B-cells produce cytokines, substances that attack bacteria. When T- and B-cells are suppressed, the immune system struggles to identify and destroy any pathogens invading our bodies, so we have an increased risk of infection.

Alcohol Can Exacerbate Cellulite

While alcohol isn't a cause of cellulite, it can make it worse. The toxins it contains can contribute to the build-up of unsightly "orange-peel" skin. Booze encourages fluid retention and increases fatty deposits in areas such as your thighs, stomach, arms and bottom. The calories in alcohol are also a cause of weight gain, which can lead to dimply skin. Another component is dehydration (which your Sahara-dry mouth after a night on the booze will tell you is a side effect). As our bodies are normally around 55–65 per cent water, not having enough means that the kidneys, liver and digestive system fail to eliminate toxins satisfactorily, leading to fat accumulation just beneath the skin. This is hard for the body to metabolize, which can contribute to the puckered "cottage cheese" texture of cellulite. Glass of water, anyone?

Your Sex Life Can Go from Sizzle to Fizzle

Although drinking alcohol may increase your desire for sex, that doesn't mean you'll have good sex. In fact, it could be downright disappointing. For men, in the short term, the inability to maintain an erection can put a dampener on things; in the long term, full-on impotence may occur. Women may experience reduced lubrication and find it harder to reach orgasm. If they do get there, the experience is likely to be less intense than if they'd been sober. Balance and coordination are negatively affected by booze, meaning a sexual encounter may be a clumsy fumble. For both men and women, alcohol reduces sexual sensitivity and satisfaction.

But what if it's not just disappointment you have to contend with? What if it's something more sinister? Alcohol reduces inhibitions and impairs our judgement. When drunk, you may take risks you wouldn't normally take – like having unprotected sex.

Fertility Can Be Affected

Alcohol can reduce fertility in both men and women. Research has shown that if a woman drinks between one and five alcoholic beverages a week, her chances of conceiving are reduced; having ten or more drinks a week further reduces the odds. Even drinking lightly can increase the time it takes to get pregnant, as alcohol affects ovulation and menstrual cycles. Women who drink seven drinks a week (or more than three drinks on one occasion) are more likely to have irregular periods and fertility issues.

As for men, the amount they knock back will have an impact on fertility. Excessive alcohol decreases testosterone levels and makes having a low sperm count more likely. Just five alcoholic drinks a week could reduce sperm quality. Heavy drinking can also cause impotence and a reduced libido – so unless you're hoping for an immaculate conception, it's a good idea to reduce your intake or stop completely if you're hoping to hear the pitter-patter of tiny feet any time soon.

Sleep Is Disrupted

Drinking alcohol near bedtime may help us get to sleep initially, but it will affect the quality of our slumber throughout the night. Why? Drinking disrupts our sleep cycle – particularly the Rapid Eye Movement (REM) stage of sleep. REM sleep is when we dream, and it's important for mental restoration – which includes things like memory and emotional processing. If it's disrupted, our sleep is lighter and more restless, meaning we'll be drowsy, irritable and unable to concentrate properly the next day.

After drinking, sleep may also be interrupted by frequent trips to the bathroom. Besides the fact that more liquid is going into our body – so we'll need to urinate more – alcohol is a diuretic, encouraging the body to lose yet more fluid.

Causing excessive relaxation of the muscles in the head, neck and throat, alcohol can also suppress breathing and increase the risk of snoring and other sleep-disordered breathing, such as sleep apnoea. Those with alcohol in their system when in the land of nod are also more likely to sleepwalk, sleep talk and even sleep eat.

Hair Loss Can Occur

Alcoholics and heavy drinkers often can't boast a full, glossy mane. People who drink to excess generally don't focus on a well-balanced diet and obtain many of their calories from booze. But a combination of vitamins, minerals, proteins, fats and carbohydrates is vital to a healthy scalp and full head of hair. Even if a heavy drinker is eating well, alcohol can interfere with the absorption of these nutrients by irritating the stomach lining and increasing the production of acid in the digestive system.

Dehydration is another way locks, or their lustre, can be lost. Lack of water can damage follicles, making hair brittle and more likely to fall out. Dehydration can also cause dandruff. On top of this, alcohol can increase the body's production of oestrogen, fluctuating levels of which have been linked to hair loss. Stress is another factor related to hair thinning. And stress can be caused by exhaustion, which is often the result of not sleeping well. And, yep, not getting good-quality sleep is a consequence of drinking too much alcohol.

Booze Shrinks Your Brain

It probably comes as no surprise that alcoholics and heavy drinkers are damaging their brains. Studies have found that their brains are smaller and lighter than the brains of people who are not alcoholics. But did you know that even a moderate amount of alcohol will cause your brain to shrivel? Any alcohol consumption can impair brain volume and function, and drinkers are more likely to suffer from conditions like hippocampal atrophy. This is a disorder identified by the decline of the hippocampus (a major component of the brain, thought to be the centre of emotion, learning, memory and the autonomic nervous system). The brain shrinkage caused by excessive drinking affects the brain's "wiring", which means that the communication between different regions of the brain is hindered. Hello, confusion!

Acid Reflux Is Aggravated

If you suffer from acid reflux – where acidic gastric fluid flows into the oesophagus, resulting in heartburn, pain and nausea – alcohol can aggravate this in a few ways:

- Alcohol relaxes the lower oesophageal sphincter, which allows the contents of the stomach to leak into the oesophagus.
- Drinking makes your stomach produce more acid than it usually would, which can cause inflammation and irritation of the delicate stomach lining. Drinks with higher alcohol content – like hard liquors – are more likely to trigger reflux than drinks such as beer or wine.
- After you've had a few drinks, you are more likely to opt for unhealthy foods of the fried and fatty variety, which can worsen acid reflux by relaxing the lower oesophageal sphincter.

Acid reflux can progress into a more severe condition called gastro-oesophageal reflux disease (GERD), with symptoms other than heartburn, such as the regurgitation of food, difficulty swallowing, coughing, wheezing and chest pain.

Drinking Comes at a Cost

Along with making our heads lighter, drinking makes our wallets lighter, too. But it's not just the price of that fancy cocktail or that bottle of Chardonnay that has you wearing out your debit card – there are hidden costs of drinking that you may not have even considered. A study revealed that 18–35-year-olds in the UK are frequently spending more than they intend after drinking, which adds up to £1,400 (US $1,850) a year. According to the survey, they are spending an extra £340 (US $450) a year on fast food they regret eating the next day, £280 (US $370) on taxis when they had intended to catch public transport home and £174 (US $230) on impromptu rounds of shots. Drunkenness can also lead to expensive carelessness – the poll showed that 27 per cent of Brits have smashed their phone on a night out, 19 per cent have lost jewellery, 26 per cent have ruined a pricey item of clothing, 9 per cent have misplaced their handbag and 8 per cent have even lost their shoes.

Alcohol Impairs Eyesight

The health of your eyes can be affected by drinking in a number of ways. Problems include itchiness, irritation and fluctuation in acuity, such as blurring or double/distorted vision. Alcohol swells the blood vessels in the eyes, which makes them look bloodshot and red. Associated swelling or inflammation can cause the eyelids to twitch and bring about an increased sensitivity to light. Rapid eye movement – an involuntary movement back and forth – can also occur. Colours can become distorted when drinking due to the fact that alcohol decreases the reaction time of the pupils, meaning they are unable to dilate or constrict when reacting to light levels, which hinders the ability to see contrasting colours or different shades of the same colour. While these might seem like minor problems, long-term heavy drinking can permanently damage the optic nerves, which send visual information from the eyes to the brain. Heavy drinkers are more prone to eye conditions and declining eyesight. Toxic amblyopia is the term used to describe permanent loss of vision caused by a toxin, such as alcohol.

Alcohol Harms Your Gut Health

Drinking too much alcohol can make it harder for your body to digest food and absorb nutrients, especially vitamins and proteins. Why? Booze reduces the amount of digestive enzymes the pancreas produces to help us break down what we've eaten. Drinking too much can cause stomach pain and diarrhoea but also more serious digestive problems such as dysbiosis – a condition that occurs when the bacteria in your gastrointestinal tract becomes unbalanced. In essence, the "bad" gut bacteria multiply and push out the "good" bacteria that are vital for a healthy gut. Alcohol – particularly sweet wines, ciders, cocktails and liqueurs – contains sugar, and consuming a lot of sugar messes with the balance of your gut bacteria. While spirits are usually low in sugar, mixers often aren't – a 250 ml (8½ fl. oz) can of gin and tonic contains 3½ teaspoons of sugar. Something to bear in mind during your next trip to the bar.

NOTHING GOOD
EVER HAPPENS IN
A BLACKOUT. I'VE
NEVER WOKEN
UP AND BEEN
LIKE, "WHAT IS
THIS PILATES MAT
DOING OUT?"

AMY SCHUMER

Cutting Down

One in three Americans admit they drink too much, while around a quarter of Britons want to cut back their intake of alcohol. The reasons are varied and could involve any one or a combination of the following: to be healthier, to save money, to sleep better, to have more energy, to lose weight, to allow your brain to fire on all cylinders, or simply to live hangover-free. Some say the rising trend to drink less is being led by the millennial generation, who are increasingly opting for soft drinks in a bid to remain healthy, secure future employment (who wants their potential boss to see them chugging from a beer bong on social media?) and stay in control. Many millennials see getting drunk as "something done by an older generation", with 40 per cent in one survey describing it as "pathetic" or "embarrassing". Ouch! Whatever your reasons for wanting to drink less, this chapter will offer advice, guidance and support to help you on your way.

Write Down Your Reasons

A big first step in reducing your alcohol intake is to write down an "intention statement" – for example, "I intend to cut back on my drinking" or "I'll stop at one glass of wine". Intention statements can increase your accountability and offer a focus to your goals. Next, write down *why* you are deciding to drink less – perhaps you want to feel healthier, improve your relationships or start training for a physical challenge. The act of writing down both your aims and your reasons – and seeing them in black and white – will help to motivate you to achieve success. You could even pin these reasons up somewhere in your house (in the drinks cabinet or on the wine rack, perhaps) to remind you why you've decided to cut back.

Tell People

If you tell your family and friends that you've decided to cut back your drinking, they will be able to offer you support. They'll know not to pour you another drink when your glass is empty and will be on hand to give you a pep talk if they see your resolve waning. Even better, why not encourage someone to join you on your "drink-less journey"? Being accountable to someone who has the same goal as you means you can help each other stick to the plan. Making your intentions known more widely might help, too. Telling people on social media that you plan to drink less will encourage you to do it. The more people who know, the more people there will be to celebrate with you when you succeed, or to prove wrong if they doubted you.

Find an Alternative Coping Strategy

Do you use booze as a crutch, drinking when you're lonely, angry, worried or perhaps simply because you've had a tough day at work? Drinking to deal with stress is common, but, as alcohol is a depressant, it can often make things worse – your thoughts and emotions may be left in a downward spiral. Instead of boozing when you're feeling anxious, find new, healthy ways to cope when you feel like reaching for a drink. Perhaps try the following to lift your spirits:

- Go for a walk or run
- Call a friend
- Listen to your favourite song
- Watch your favourite film or TV show
- Look at photos that make you smile
- Draw or paint something
- Cook something delicious

Drink the Same, Reduce the Alcohol

Opt for drinks with low or reduced alcohol content. "Low-alcohol drinks" are beverages that have an alcoholic strength by volume (ABV) of between 0.5 and 1.2 per cent. "Reduced-alcohol drinks" have an alcohol content lower than the average strength of a particular drink. Assuming you still have the same number of drinks, choosing these options can help you to stay within the recommended drinking guidelines. Substituting your regular tipple with one lower in alcohol is an easy and sustainable approach to cutting down your drinking. So, if you go for a glass of wine after work, you will more than halve the number of units you drink by swapping the usual 12–14 per cent for a 5.5 per cent one. Over time, this will reduce the risk of undesirable health implications caused by drinking too much.

Keep Track with an App

Download an app to help you keep track of your drinking. They can do everything from calculating the units and calories you consume, to reviewing your drinking habits over time, plus offering support and motivation. Here are just a few that may be useful:

- **Drink Less** allows you to complete a daily mood diary to understand the effects of hangovers, offers games to strengthen your resolve to drink less, creates plans to prepare for tricky situations and outlines exercises to help change your relationship with alcohol.
- **Drink Free Days** lets you nominate the days you want to give drinking a miss, then offers practical daily support, tips and reminders to help you stick to your plan.
- **Drinks Meter** compares your drinking to that of your peers and offers a "what you think about your drinking vs. where you really are" feature, as well as outlining calorie equivalents and health information.

Change Venue

Sometimes you may end up in a pub or bar by default. "Fancy a drink?" rolls off the tongue so naturally for some people that it may not even occur to them that there are other options. But there are! Instead of hanging out in bars all the time, learn how to "soberlize" by meeting friends, family and colleagues in other establishments, like coffee shops, tearooms, smoothie bars, restaurants, ice-cream parlours, milkshake shops or even alcohol-free bars (yes, they do exist). While you're mixing up *where* you meet, why not also mix up *what time* you meet? Breakfast and brunch meet-ups don't carry as much expectation to drink as, say, dinner. And if you're watching a sporting event, invite friends over to your place – you'll almost certainly drink less than you would at a bar surrounded by drunk people.

Be Mindful

Research has shown that as little as 11 minutes of meditation – or mindfulness training – could help heavy drinkers to cut back on their alcohol consumption. Those involved in the study carried out by researchers at University College London found themselves drinking 9.3 units of alcohol (the equivalent to around three pints of beer) less than usual over the following week. They listened to audio recordings encouraging mindfulness, a technique which focuses one's awareness on the present moment by thinking consciously about one's feelings, thoughts, bodily sensations and – more specifically in this study – cravings for alcohol. The recordings told them to acknowledge their cravings so that they would become more tolerable as temporary events, without the need to act on the urge to drink. Practising mindfulness makes a person more aware of their impulse to give in to cravings – people are less likely to reach for a drink automatically if they're consciously aware of their hankering. There are many websites, apps and books that can help you to become more mindful.

Pimp Your Drink

You're at the bar and you've ordered a glass of wine. The bartender asks, "Large or small glass?" You panic. You want a large glass but you've promised yourself you'll drink less. What to do? Turn your white wine into a spritzer! Ask the bartender to use lemonade or soda water as a mixer, then relax and enjoy your *large* glass of wine (that's really a small). Or do like the Spanish and go for some *calimocho*, which is red wine mixed with cola. If you use half a small glass of wine (about 60 ml or 2 fl. oz), there will be less than one unit of alcohol per glass.

Cook with Leftover Wine

A half-drunk bottle of wine sitting on the side can be all too tempting. You may polish it off even when you don't really want it just because it's *there*. But you don't have to drink every last drop – you could cook with the leftovers. Wine that has been open for a few days and is perhaps past its prime is great for cooking or using in salad dressings and marinades. Old wine is perfect for deglazing a pan and making a quick sauce or gravy, as well as boosting the flavour of stews, soups and casseroles. If you know you won't be cooking for a while after opening a bottle of wine, you could always freeze any remaining wine in an ice-cube tray to use in cooking as and when you need it. Remember, though, that alcohol doesn't entirely "cook off", so it still counts as part of your overall intake.

Give Rounds a Miss

It's so easy to get sucked into buying rounds of drinks. Even if you only want to stay for one, you may feel obliged to get involved in the round for fear of seeming rude, cheap or "not part of the gang". When you're trying to cut back on drinking, the round is a dangerous thing. Not only will you try to keep up with the fastest drinker in the group, you'll most likely stay longer in the pub than you intended, either waiting for it to be your turn to buy drinks or waiting for everyone who "owes" you a drink to buy their round. You'll most likely drink more than you planned, as well as spending more. Don't buy in to rounds, even if you feel uncomfortable saying no at first – or just do smaller rounds with a couple of friends.

Adapt Your Routine

We are creatures of habit. We know what we like and like what we know. Veering from our regular patterns – our comfort zone – can feel daunting and positively unappealing. But, when it comes to your drinking patterns, stepping away from what you normally do may be the only way to cut down. Let's say, for example, you usually come home from work and pour yourself a glass of wine – how about you prepare yourself a different, non-alcoholic drink instead? Or maybe you always head to the pub after work on a Friday – why not suggest to friends that you meet somewhere else (for dim sum, to go bowling, or any place where drinking isn't the primary activity)? Mixing things up and resetting your habits and routines will stop your brain from looking forward to what it's expecting (booze) so that it will come to expect the unexpected!

Get the Gear

If you mix your own drinks at home, the "free pour" is a dangerous method when you're trying to cut back on your alcohol intake. You may think you're pouring yourself a single but it could, in fact, be a triple! To combat this and find a way to drink in moderation, use one or all of these bartending tools when mixing yourself a drink:

- **A jigger spirit measure –** This hourglass-shaped device will allow you to measure out single and double shots.
- **A mini angled measuring cup –** A tool to measure the amount of alcohol you pour. The angled surface means you can read the measurements from above.
- **A wine measure –** These are often made out of stainless steel and can be purchased in a few sizes, usually 125 ml, 175 ml and 250 ml.
- **A pour spout –** Designed to replace the cap on a bottle of liquor, this spout will allow you to measure an accurate and consistent amount of alcohol.

Take Wine Off the Table

If you like to have a glass of wine with dinner, make sure that it stays *a glass* by removing the bottle from the dining table. If you keep it there, it's staring you in the face, calling out "Drink me", and chances are you'll top yourself up – or someone else will – when your glass becomes empty, or nearly empty, until the bottle runs out. To stop this from happening, pour yourself a glass, then cork the bottle and put it away and out of sight. Instead, keep a jug of water on the table. If something is within easy reach, it's likely you're going to, you know, reach for it. Take the half-drunk bottle of wine out of the equation and it doesn't become an option.

THE RULE IS
SIMPLE: BE
SOBER AND
TEMPERATE,
AND YOU WILL
BE HEALTHY.

BENJAMIN FRANKLIN

Stopping Completely

In 2019, as many as 4 million people in the UK tried to give up alcohol for January. Some people embark on such a challenge with a view to give up only in the short-term – vowing to abstain from drinking for Dry January, give it up for Lent or "Go Sober for October". The Dry January campaign was first launched in 2013 and, since then, things are looking promising: more than half of those taking part complete the entire month, and most are drinking less overall six months later.

Some people want to banish booze from their life for longer periods or even for life. They may recognize their drinking habits as being unhealthy – or addictive – and want to take control. This chapter is split into two sections – "Stopping for Short Periods" and "Stopping for Longer Periods or Life" – and offers advice on how to achieve these goals. No one's promising it'll be easy, but if you stick to your guns and harness all your willpower, it'll be worth it. You can do it – and you'll be glad you did.

STOPPING FOR SHORT PERIODS

Sign Up for a Challenge

Rather than just telling yourself you're not going to drink, actively seek out a challenge where other people know what you're doing so you'll be more accountable. If you quit your mission to give up, these people will know about it, so you'll be more likely to stick to your intentions. Here are a couple of challenges you can commit to:

- **One Year No Beer** has more than 25,000 members in 90 countries and offers guidance, daily videos, training in fitness, diet and mindset, and an online support network to encourage you to complete their 28-day, 90-day or 365-day challenge. The focus is on building new habits and creating a new mindset when it comes to alcohol. **(www.oneyearnobeer.com)**
- **James Swanwick's 30-Day No-Alcohol Challenge** sees James explaining how a photo of him with Jennifer Aniston prompted him to give up booze. He went from "fat and broke to hosting SportsCenter on ESPN" and now runs a programme to help others achieve life-changing results through not drinking. **(www.30daynoalcoholchallenge.com)**

Show Me the Money

A bottle of wine here, a round in the pub there... The amount we spend on booze can quickly add up. In fact, the average person in Britain spends around £787 (US $1,008) a year on alcohol, which amounts to a whopping £50,000 (US $64,000) throughout their lifetime. Americans are estimated to spend about 1 per cent of their gross annual income on alcohol. And it's not just the cost of the booze we need to consider. When we drink, we lose our spending inhibitions, so we end up saying, "What the hell!" and reaching for our credit card more readily.

Each time you choose not to have a drink, put aside the money you would have spent. Then at the end of the month use it to treat yourself to something that will give you more lasting pleasure and value than booze, and without the negative side effects.

Avoid Boozy Events

Oscar Wilde knew what he was talking about when he said, "I can resist anything except temptation." If you were trying to lose weight, you wouldn't plonk a giant, gooey chocolate cake in front of yourself, would you? So, why, if you're trying to give up alcohol, would you put yourself in a scenario where you're likely to be tempted to drink? During the period you want to remain sober, try to avoid events or social outings where booze will be flowing freely. You can still have a social life, but you may just have to reframe it temporarily. Meet friends in cafes rather than bars, and say no to certain invitations (that's allowed!). If you're really serious about abstaining from alcohol, don't put yourself in temptation's way. Of course, it's not realistic to avoid all boozy events forever – unless you don't want to go to your best friend's wedding or celebrate your dad's 70th – but if steering clear of occasions that will weaken your willpower for a while is the only way to achieve your goal, so be it.

Be the Designated Driver

There are a few concrete reasons why you definitely *can't* drink – you're pregnant, you're on antibiotics, for religious reasons or you're training for a physical challenge. Another non-negotiable one is that you're driving. If your car is parked outside, it's not even on your radar to drink because *you can't*. And if temptation does strike, the thought of paying for a taxi home and then returning to retrieve your vehicle in the morning will likely be enough to quash the allure of the bottle. There are other advantages of driving on a night out, too. You'll be able to give your friends a lift home, which will earn you their respect and goodwill when you next need a favour. On the flipside, you can make a quick getaway if your friends are getting drunk and you're really not enjoying their slurred regalings of That Time When.

Use the Same Glass for a Different Drink

The power of the mind is a wonderful thing. "Trick" yourself into thinking you're drinking an alcoholic beverage by using the glass your usual drink would be served in. Flavoured sparkling water in a wine glass; a tonic and lime in a highball tumbler; a mocktail in a martini glass... There's something more satisfying about having a drink from a nice glass – like eating from a china plate rather than a plastic one. And if you don't want to answer any annoying questions as to why you're not drinking, the people you're with will probably assume that what you've got is alcoholic given the glass you're using. Deceptive? Perhaps. Effective? Absolutely!

Switch Your Drink

Opt for the non-alcoholic equivalent of your tipple of choice. There's so much choice these days for teetotallers. Gone are the days when an orange juice or Coke would be the only vaguely appealing options. Now, there's a huge number of non-alcoholic drinks on the market. There's non-alcoholic beer, non-alcoholic wine, even non-alcoholic spirits. If cocktails are more your thing, there are countless mocktails being shaken up that taste just as delicious as their alcoholic counterparts. Need some inspiration? Turn to page 107 to check out some Booze-Free Beverages.

Identify Your Triggers

What are the triggers that tempt you to drink? Perhaps it's setting foot in a pub? Maybe it's hanging out with "Crazy Karen"? Or it could be sitting down for a session of Face-stalking on your social media? Whatever it is that will have your mouth watering for a chilled bottle of beer or a glass of full-bodied red, avoid it at all costs during the time you've set aside to be teetotal. Why put yourself in a position that will make things harder for you? If you can't readily identify your triggers, sit down and think back to the last five times you drank. Is there a common denominator? Perhaps you drank at the same time on each occasion, like after work. Maybe you were with the same group of people – your "boozy" friends. Or possibly the venue was the same – your local that you walk past on the way home. Once you know exactly what you need to avoid in order to resist temptation, it'll be that much easier.

Load Up on Nutrients

Alcohol saps your body of vitamins and minerals that are vital for good health. Give your body a helping hand to replenish them.

- **Vitamin A –** This helps with cell growth and keeping the immune system in good working order. Stock up on dairy products, meat (especially liver), fish, carrots, broccoli, apricots and leafy greens.
- **B1 (thiamine**) **–** Very important for your eyes and brain, thiamine can be found in cauliflower, beans, carrots, rice, nuts and wheat.
- **B2 (riboflavin) –** This helps with metabolism and other cell functions, and is present in eggs, lean meats, low-fat milk, asparagus, spinach and fortified cereals.
- **B6 (pyridoxine) –** A depletion of B6 can lead to anaemia, depression and cognitive dysfunction. Have a better chance of avoiding these conditions by consuming potatoes, bananas, poultry and prune juice.
- **Vitamin C –** Essential for bone and tissue repair, vitamin C also eliminates free radicals (which can cause cancer). Citrus fruits, berries, tomatoes and kale are all good sources.

- **Vitamin D –** A lack of vitamin D can cause issues with your bones and teeth. Find it in fish, dairy products, liver and through exposure to sunlight.
- **Vitamin E –** If you are deficient in vitamin E, you may become disoriented and have vision problems. It can also lead to muscle weakness. To combat this, load up on whole grains, sunflower seeds, spinach and nut oils.
- **Vitamin K –** Deficiencies are rare but they can result in your blood not clotting. Opt for meat, eggs, liver and fish.
- **Calcium –** Important for good bone and teeth health, calcium is in dairy products, leafy green vegetables, tofu and nuts.
- **Zinc –** Zinc deficiency affects the gastrointestinal tract, skin, central nervous system and reproductive systems, as well as causing hair loss, diarrhoea and acne. Shellfish, legumes, whole grains and avocados are high in zinc .
- **Iron –** A lack of iron can lead to anaemia, which results in tiredness, heart palpitations, pale skin and shortness of breath. Baked potatoes, cashew nuts, tofu and spinach are all iron-rich.
- **Magnesium –** Fatigue, muscle cramps, osteoporosis and an irregular heartbeat are symptoms of deficiency. Bananas, tuna, kale and asparagus are good sources.

Manage Withdrawal Symptoms

Often when people quit something for a short period, they go cold turkey. People may go on benders over the Christmas period then, come the New Year, they say, "Right, no more booze!" If you do this, prepare yourself for the fact that your body and mind will be in for a shock. Quitting suddenly can affect you in a number of ways, including poor concentration, fatigue, sweating, shaking, headaches, difficulty sleeping, nausea and a lack of appetite. Some of the more serious side effects can include fever, confusion and even hallucinations. If you experience any concerning side effects in the first week of giving up alcohol, you may want to speak to your doctor to see if they can prescribe anything to help. However, if you want to ride out the side effects and deal with them naturally, it's important to drink lots of water, eat a balanced diet, exercise regularly and see friends and family often.

Just Say No

It sounds easy enough to use the word "no" – one of the simplest, shortest words in the dictionary – but, in reality, it can be very difficult. The other hard part about saying no is actually meaning it. If someone offers you a drink and you reply with, "Um... well... er... no", there's a high chance that they will clock your wavering and return from the bar with a G&T for you. "But, I said no," you'll feebly protest, and they'll say, "Yeah, but you didn't really *mean* it." And then, just like that, temptation is in front of you and you're off the wagon. If someone offers you a drink, say "No thanks" quickly and firmly so that you don't give yourself time to change your mind – and you don't give the person an opportunity to tell you what you actually want. It's your body, your decision and your prerogative to decline.

STOPPING FOR LONGER PERIODS OR LIFE

Seek Help

If you think that you may have an addiction to alcohol, it's important to get some professional help – perhaps in the form of an addiction counsellor. Kicking an addiction isn't easy, and attempting to do it alone is not only unrealistic but also potentially dangerous. You'll face barriers, setbacks and, sometimes, brick walls. You'll experience emotions that have either long been buried – drowned out by the booze – or that you've never even felt before. An addiction counsellor can equip you with the tools required to deal with the scary unknown so that you can persevere through the dark days, making you less likely to reach for the bottle. Depending on your location and circumstances, try speaking first to your doctor or seeking out relevant advice and resources online or at a local library or health centre.

Exercise

Exercising is a highly effective tool when trying to kick a bad habit or overcome an addiction. When you drink, your brain releases dopamine, a chemical that is associated with rewarding behaviours. When you exercise, dopamine is also released – along with serotonin and endorphins – which means you'll get the same "buzz" from working out as you did from a bottle of wine, with a much better outcome for your health. Exercise activates the brain's "pleasure centres" in a positive rather than negative way. Exercise has also been found to reduce cravings – just 10 minutes of physical exertion can crush a craving for alcohol.

Exercise occupies your time, mind and energy – if you're pounding the pavement or zooming up and down a pool, you're not sitting around feeling tempted to drink. Your focus is elsewhere, namely on smashing your workout goals. Studies on recovering alcoholics have found that including daily exercise in their treatment programme greatly increases the likelihood of them staying sober; those who do not keep active are much more likely to relapse.

Exercise has also been shown to help the brain recover from alcohol abuse, literally rebuilding the brain tissue that's been lost. Aerobic exercise can generate new neurons, improving your ability to learn and boosting your memory. When you stop drinking, an exercise programme is also one of the best stress busters around, able to boost your mood and fight off negative feelings. Getting active also increases your physical fitness, confidence and self-esteem, which can only be a positive thing when you're trying to combat the gruelling "I need a drink" days.

It may be a good idea to hire a personal trainer to jump-start your training programme and keep you motivated when you first give up alcohol. Not only will they make you accountable, they'll also be able to devise an appropriate fitness plan for you, taking into account your capabilities.

Ultimately, if you replace the time you would have spent drinking with doing exercise, you'll soon realize how much more your body is capable of and how much booze was previously holding you back.

Join a Sober Community

There is so much help out there when it comes to quitting booze. The trick is to find the thing that works for you. Here are a few routes you could take on your journey to Soberville:

- **Alcoholics Anonymous (AA) –** The most widely known alcohol support group, AA is an international organization that encourages alcoholics to share their experiences with each other via the attendance of meetings. It also uses a "12-step programme" as a means of reaching sobriety.
- **SMART Recovery –** The SMART Recovery approach is scientifically based and uses cognitive behavioural therapy (CBT) and motivational enhancement therapy (MET) to get results. The programme highlights four areas in the process of banishing booze: building motivation, coping with urges, problem solving and lifestyle balance.
- **Refuge Recovery –** Based on Buddhist principles, Refuge Recovery uses mindfulness, compassion, generosity and forgiveness to heal the pain of addiction.

Keep Your Home Booze-Free

Don't keep alcohol in your house. Get rid of the half-drunk bottles of spirits, avoid stocking up on wine... and that sticky bottle of something from Christmas at the back of your cupboard? Pour it away! If it's not there, you can't drink it. If you're at home and there's alcohol within easy reach, it's more likely your willpower will wane and you'll find yourself caving in to the craving. If there's an obstacle between you and booze – i.e. the need to go out and buy some first – you're far less likely to give in. If you're worried that a single obstacle won't deter you, create several barriers for yourself. When you arrive home, change into slouchy "wouldn't be seen dead in public" clothes so you'd need to change to leave the house. Or wash your hair so you'd have to dry it before venturing outside. If fulfilling your craving for a drink becomes a hassle, you're more likely not to bother.

Feed Your Sugar Cravings

A small glass of wine can contain 2–3 per cent of your daily intake of sugar, and a cocktail or a spirit with a sugary mixer can have a huge 60 per cent. If you're a heavy drinker and you stop drinking, your blood-sugar level will drop, meaning you're likely to have a craving for something sugary-sweet. You may also get sugar cravings because you're no longer getting the serotonin boost that alcohol provides to make you feel good, and sugar can be an appealing substitute for this. Go with it – at least temporarily. Although it's not a good idea to trade one addiction (alcohol) for another (sugar), while you're in the initial stages of trying to cut booze from your life, save your willpower for refusing alcohol. Don't beat yourself up if you eat two bowls of ice cream or if you take an extra handful of gummy bears.

Read About Quitting

There are two main reasons why reading up on how to stop drinking can be beneficial: one, you'll learn a lot; and two, you'll feel less alone. People who write about kicking habits are often professionals like psychologists, doctors and counsellors, or recovering addicts themselves. People who have been there, done that, bought the T-shirt (and written the book) have a wealth of great advice and wise words that will help you on your journey to a sober life. Some books that may be helpful and relatable include:

* *Dry* by Augusten Burroughs (2003)
* *The Unexpected Joy of Being Sober* by Catherine Gray (2017)
* *Blackout* by Sarah Hepola (2015)
* *The Sober Diaries* by Claire Pooley (2017)
* *The Easy Way to Control Alcohol* by Allen Carr (2009)
* *Clean* by David Sheff (2014)

Look After Yourself

When you're drinking heavily, you're often in self-destruct mode. You've stopped caring about consequences and can be your own worst enemy. Now that you've stopped drinking, you must be kinder to yourself. Before, all you "needed" was a drink. Now, you need a whole plethora of things and it's up to you to make sure you get them. If you're tired, sleep. If you're hungry, eat. If you're smelly, wash. If you're sad, call a friend. If your brain is buzzing, meditate. If you're feeling cooped up, get some fresh air. Whatever you need, try to find the solution – preferably not at the bottom of a wine or beer bottle. It's OK to handle yourself with kid gloves for a while. Giving up drinking is hard; don't make it harder by neglecting your needs. You deserve to be well looked after, so bring on the age of self-care.

Keep Busy

If you're in the initial stages of trying to kick a habit, sitting still is often one of the worst things you can do. It'll give you time to think, "I really want a drink right now... I'm bored. A drink would entertain me... Just one won't hurt..." Don't sit and think; get up and do something to distract yourself and quash those cravings. Like what? Anything! Try one or all of these things:

- Do some exercise
- Clean your home
- Clear your junk mail
- Alphabetize your book collection
- Read
- Declutter
- Bake something
- Fix your split seams or sew on your popped-off buttons
- Watch TV
- Do a jigsaw puzzle
- Knit
- Play solitaire
- Do a crossword

Realize that Booze Doesn't Define Fun

As a society, we often associate fun activities with drinking. Going to a show... Having a barbecue... Watching sport... Eating in a fancy restaurant... Chilling by the pool... Binge-watching Netflix... All of these things are enhanced with a drink in your hand, right? Well, actually, no. It's time we stopped giving alcohol so much credit for the fun we have. Going to shows, spending time with friends, eating delicious food and vegging out to your favourite film are all fun activities in themselves. You may have just got so used to booze tagging along that you assume it's the "fun-maker". But these things will still be fun – perhaps even more so – without alcohol muscling in on the action.

Go Outside

There's a lot to be said for the healing powers of nature. Being outside – and even looking at images of the great outdoors – has been shown to reduce anger, fear, anxiety, depression and stress – some or all of which you might be battling separately while also desperately craving a drink. It's not just your emotional well-being that increases when you're exposed to nature: your physical well-being gets a boost, too. Blood pressure is reduced, muscle tension is lessened, your immune system is improved and inflammation is diminished. Fresh air, forests, birds chirping, rivers, sunshine, mountains, flowers, hills, parks and all that Mother Nature has to offer are such powerful tools to combat alcohol addiction that nature-based therapies are now growing in availability and popularity. Wilderness therapy – also known as outdoor therapy – uses the outdoors to help people in their recovery. So, immerse yourself in nature whenever you can and be mindful of what you're seeing, hearing, smelling and feeling.

Remind Yourself that You're in Charge

If you're craving a drink, the thought of it – pouring it out, bringing the glass to your mouth, feeling the cool liquid slide down your throat, the warming sensation that spreads through your body – can become all-consuming. Your thoughts – "Need a drink... Want a drink... Must have a drink..." – can control your actions and convince you that everything will be terrible unless you have that drink. But a thought can't control your hand. Only you can. And if you want your hand to *not* reach for a drink, then don't allow your thoughts to treat you like a hapless puppet. Of course, when you're fighting an addiction, this is easier said than done, which is why you may have to give yourself pep talks along the way. Remind yourself of everything you're doing right, congratulate yourself on the small victories, tell yourself that you deserve to be happy – you deserve to be sober.

Form a Teetotal Tribe

Having an addiction can be very lonely. You can be so locked inside your own head, and so tunnel-visioned on where your next drink is coming from, that your relationships take a battering. Then there's the denial, the guilt, the shame and the self-hate that you try to deal with alone. But once you've decided to be sober, you can work on rebuilding your existing relationships – and, perhaps more importantly, forging new ones. You may find new friendships through the channels you take to quit, such as AA meetings, meet-up groups and online support groups. The people in your new sober squad will understand what you're going through. You can lean on each other when the going gets tough and tell each other when you want to drink. Then you can celebrate each other's non-drinking milestones with gusto – your teetotal troops will truly understand the significance of each anniversary, just as you will with theirs. When it comes to staying sober, there's safety in numbers.

Own Your Decision

Have confidence in your decision not to drink. Don't feel like you have to explain in great detail why you're not drinking to whomever you're with. When asked what you'd like to have, don't use "just" as a prefix – "Just a tonic water, please" – because it makes it sound like you need to justify your decision. Some people feel uneasy if they're drinking without someone else to "keep them company". That's their problem. Don't allow their insecurities to impact your drinking habits and lure you into adding a shot of gin to your tonic. The more confident you become with your commitment to banish booze from your life, the less strange it will feel to be The One Not Drinking. Before long, people will accept your decision and stop with the raised eyebrows, nosy questions and attempts to weaken your resolve.

LESS ALCOHOL =
MORE ENERGY,
MORE HEALTH,
MORE RELAXED,
MORE TIME,
MORE MONEY.

JAMES SWANWICK

Life After Alcohol

The benefits of cutting back or giving up alcohol are so abundant that it might just fit into the "Why didn't I do this sooner?" category – along with letting go of grudges and figuring out exactly what you can and can't recycle. Like with anything in life that tips from fun and moderate to "I need to get a handle on this", as soon as you do ditch the drink you'll likely breathe a huge sigh of relief. Yes, there may be days when you miss that boozy buzz, but if alcohol was beginning to dominate your life, you can now be free from its clutches. You'll feel better, look better, act better, work better, sleep better and generally be better. Your wallet will be heavier and your heart will be lighter – no more hangovers, hangxiety or "Hang on, where did I leave my bag?" freak-outs. This chapter explores how not drinking could improve your life, then hears from those who have been there, done that, spilt beer down their T-shirt and decided to call time on their drinking.

You'll Be More Balanced

When you're drinking, your mind doesn't fire on all cylinders. Your reactions, your ability to reason, your capacity to make good decisions and your ability to work out day-to-day issues are dulled and fuzzy. Team this with an unpredictable set of emotions – one minute you're joyously happy, the next you're in a depressed funk – and it's likely you didn't know if you were coming or going when alcohol was part of your life. You could have felt unbalanced, erratic and, frankly, out of your depth. But now alcohol has been relegated to the sidelines of your life, mental clarity and emotional balance can be restored. You'll be more rational, more able to weigh up the pros and cons of a situation to figure out the best course of action. You'll interact with the world in a more level-headed, practical manner. Your sharpness will be restored and you'll be a better, more composed version of yourself.

You'll Sleep Better

When you stop drinking, one of the first things you may notice about yourself is that you'll have revived energy levels. One of the reasons for this is that you'll be getting more, better-quality sleep. Drinking alcohol disrupts your sleep cycle and you spend less time in the REM (rapid eye movement) phase of sleep. We're supposed to have between four and six cycles of REM slumber per night, but when we've been drinking we typically only achieve one or two.

Better sleep brings many benefits. You'll be more productive, you'll be able to control your emotions better, your behaviour will improve, your enthusiasm for things will heighten, your concentration will be sharpened and, above all, you'll be happier (sleep deprivation has been linked to depression). You'll also be more in control of what you eat and therefore what you weigh. This is because sleep helps to balance the hormones that control feelings of hunger and being sated.

You'll Have More Money

Whether you're a cheap-cider drinker or more of a high-end vodka kind of tippler, there's no denying that alcohol is, basically, a waste of money. You hand over your cash, knock the stuff back and then have nothing to show for it. And let's not even mention the extra costs of fast food at the end of the night and taxis to get home. Imagine how much more flush you're going to be now you've kicked booze to the curb. Whether you choose to save the money for something big – a holiday, a car – or treat yourself along the way, your wallet is going to feel the good effects, and so will you. The average spend on alcohol in the UK per week is £15 (US $20). In one month, here's what you could be enjoying instead of buying booze:

- One week: £15 (US $20) = a new book (plus a coffee to enjoy while reading it)
- Two weeks: £30 (US $40) = lunch for two
- Three weeks: £45 (US $60) = gym membership for a month
- Four weeks: £60 (US $80) = two tickets to a gig or show

Your Brain Will Repair

Alcohol is addictive because of the way it affects your brain. It resets the brain's "wiring", and if you become addicted, your brain will tell you that alcohol is the solution to whatever you need, whether it's to calm down due to stress or give you confidence in social scenarios, and so on. The more you use alcohol in such situations, the more you conclude that "alcohol is what I need". This message becomes encoded in the habit-forming part of your brain. Eventually, drinking isn't just a habit but a compulsion and coping mechanism – which can then morph into an addiction. But when you stop drinking, your brain will literally start to reconstruct, and the neural pathways that were leading to a "let's drink" conclusion will be rerouted to a "no booze for me" destination.

You'll Do Better at Work

Whether you're drinking in the middle of your workday or have a hangover from the night before, alcohol negatively impacts your work. It'll affect your judgement, concentration, coordination, reaction times, problem-solving skills, performance and, ultimately, your standard of work. This reduces productivity, which affects business objectives. Depending on your job, it's not just the bottom line that could be harmed by your drinking – your safety, and that of those around you, could also be impaired, particularly if you work with heavy machinery or you drive a vehicle.

Your drinking habits don't just affect you; they affect your colleagues, customers and clients as well. Giving up the booze means you'll be more attentive to customers and clients, and it's less likely that there will be resentment among your co-workers – they'll no longer have to mop up your mistakes or cover for you while you're dealing with a hangover. Giving up alcohol means it won't stand in the way of your professional success. Drink less, work smarter.

You'll Feel All the Feels

Depending on how much you drank, you may be surprised – or even floored – by how much you now feel without emotion-numbing alcohol coursing through your bloodstream. You'll experience *real*, undiluted emotions, rather than the emotions alcohol is dictating. If you find something funny, you'll laugh. If you find something sad, you'll cry. If you find something exciting, you'll shriek. You get the idea. Instead of life being blurry round the edges, you'll be experiencing it in HD. The world will be brighter, louder, cooler, realer. While this might seem scary – perhaps you used to drink to numb pain, stress, anxiety or any other unfavourable emotion – at least now you can focus on dealing with the thing causing these negative feelings. Drinking just masks undesirable emotions temporarily, but issues eating away at you will always catch you up. Like the saying goes: alcohol isn't the answer – it just makes you forget the question. Now you're living a sober life, your experiences will be more varied and more authentic.

You'll Be Better Hydrated

Get this: when you drink alcohol, you lose around four times as much fluid as you actually drank, because alcohol is a diuretic. So, drinking six glasses of wine is the equivalent to losing 24 glasses of water. The day after drinking alcohol, your body is dehydrated and so it will retain fluid to make up for its loss of water. Headaches are commonplace because your organs take water from the brain as they're gasping for it. Potassium and salt levels also decline, which can have an impact on nerve and muscle function, leading to nausea and fatigue. When you give up alcohol, your body will be more hydrated and less of a parched mess. Not only will your body benefit, your brain will, too. Your concentration and mood will be more stable, and the frequency with which you experience headaches will decrease.

Your Liver Function Improves

Alcohol has a negative impact on the liver. When it tries to break down the alcohol we put into our body, the chemical reaction that occurs can damage its cells. This damage can result in inflammation and scarring as the liver attempts to repair itself. If you cut out booze, your liver will start to shed the excess fat that's caused by alcohol, and liver function will begin to improve. If your liver function isn't too badly affected, it can recover within four to eight weeks. The liver plays a part in more than 500 vital functions in the body, so giving up alcohol means these processes will be vastly improved. Some of those functions include:

- Converting food nutrients for use in the body
- Helping to fight infection
- Removing contaminants
- Maintaining hormone balance
- Producing enzymes, bile and proteins
- Storing minerals and vitamins
- Regulating blood clotting
- Removing bacteria from the blood

You'll Lose Weight

When you give up alcohol, you're likely to notice weight loss within a fortnight. But it's not just the empty calories contained in alcoholic beverages that you'll be saving your body from: research has shown that drinking alcohol either before or during meals increases the amount of calories consumed – you're likely to eat more and choose less healthy, more high-fat options. You're also more likely to eat less throughout the day when alcohol is out of your life because hunger and cravings can be triggered by booze. Add to this the fact that you'll be sleeping better, so you will have more energy and be more motivated to exercise. If abstaining from alcohol is teamed with exercise, the average person could lose up to 6 kg (14 lb) of weight in a month.

Exercise Will Be More Rewarding

Alcohol and exercise are not a good combination. Consuming booze either immediately before exercising (never a good idea) or even the night before would have a hugely negative impact on your workout performance and your body. You'd feel tired more quickly because your body isn't able to eliminate properly the lactic acid you produce when you exercise, plus your power and strength would be compromised. Not to mention the fact that a hangover can cause dehydration, a headache, sickness and the shakes – which will hardly allow you to reach your PB on the treadmill. But exercising after you've given up booze means your energy levels will be soaring, your coordination won't be impaired, your reactions will be lightning-quick and your concentration will be much improved. Research has also shown that exercise can help to repair the damage your brain has suffered from drinking as well as create new neurons in your brain. On your marks... Get set... *GO!*

Your Eyes Will Sparkle

Abstaining from alcohol will positively impact the health of your peepers. Here's how:

- **The effects of dehydration will be reversed** – When your body is dehydrated, there may not be enough tears to lubricate the eyeball, causing irritation and increasing the risk of dry eye, blurred vision and infection.
- **Better sight** – High blood pressure can lead to hypertensive retinopathy, which causes damage to blood vessels in the retina, the area of the eye that allows you to focus. Cutting out alcohol means your blood pressure will be lower, safeguarding your sight.
- **Brighter, whiter eyes** – If you suffer from liver damage, the white part of your eye (sclera) can become yellow due to a build-up of old red blood cells which aren't removed by the liver. When you give up alcohol, your liver will be healthier, and your sclera will turn back from yellow to white.
- **Eye disease is less likely** – If you stop drinking, better circulation means better blood flow and oxygen supply to the eyes, warding off conditions such as glaucoma and macular degeneration.

Food Will Taste Better

When you've been drinking, your senses of taste and smell become dulled because the cells in your mouth and nose aren't functioning at full capacity. You may think that the white wine you're sipping alongside your fish is complementing the flavour of it, but actually your taste buds have been numbed. Research has found that people who consume four or more alcoholic drinks a day are more likely to experience taste impairment, compared to people who don't drink. Alcohol is an anaesthetic and can reduce the feeling in your tongue. This can affect how you perceive the texture of the food you put in your mouth. So, once you're eating without a side of taste-and-texture-numbing liquid, your food will be far more flavourful, distinctive and, ultimately, satisfying.

Your Skin Will Be Clearer

When it comes to your skin, the liver is a very important organ. As it becomes overloaded with all the toxins from alcohol, it rejects them by pushing them out through the skin, resulting in unsightly spots or full-on acne. Cocktails and beer are packed with candida, a yeast-like fungus that can cause spot breakouts. Alcohol also weakens your immune system, which means that your body can't fight off the acne-causing bacteria, which then build up in your pores. But once booze is out of your system, the positive impact on your skin will be visibly noticeable. Not only will you have fewer spots, but dandruff and eczema will also be reduced due to your skin being well hydrated. You'll also look younger. Now the toxins have been expelled, there will be a higher cell turnover and your skin will be more elastic and less wrinkly, halting any premature ageing.

Relationships Will Improve

When you were drinking heavily, chances are your moods were up and down, up and down, up and down. This was most likely exhausting, not just for you but for the people in your life – friends, family, colleagues, your partner... maybe even your pet! Perhaps they never knew where they stood with you and felt they had to tread on eggshells. There were probably arguments, disagreements, sulking, shouting, crying and – admit it – you played the victim or martyr from time to time, didn't you? Now that you're sober, all that drama will likely fall by the wayside and your relationships will change. You'll have more time and energy to invest in the people in your life, and you'll probably be a kinder, more peaceful and compassionate person, which can only be a good thing when it comes to nurturing and maintaining healthy relationships.

Sober Celebs

Take some inspiration from these teetotal stars:

- **Jennifer Lopez**, aka J-Lo, says "J-No" to drinking. The singer and actress believes booze "ruins your skin".
- Actor **Gerard Butler** avoids alcohol these days, saying, "I did a full life's worth of drinking between 14 and 27."
- Model **Tyra Banks** tried alcohol when she was 12 and decided never to drink again.
- *Sex and the City* actresses **Kim Cattrall** and **Kristin Davis** may have made the Cosmopolitan cocktail famous, but neither of them actually drinks.
- Actress and singer **Jennifer Hudson** says she's never had a drink in her life.
- *Friends* actor **Matthew Perry** struggled with alcoholism while he was filming the show, but has since decided to go sober.
- Actress **Natalie Portman** has embraced the teetotal lifestyle.
- DJ **Calvin Harris** says that since giving up alcohol, his live shows are "a million times better".

THAT'S ALL
DRUGS AND
ALCOHOL DO;
THEY CUT OFF
YOUR EMOTIONS
IN THE END.

RINGO STARR

SOBERING THOUGHTS

---

*The first-hand experiences of former drinkers are
described in the following pages. Their names
have been changed to respect their privacy.*

I stopped drinking for good three years ago. There are so many great things about being sober – waking up without a headache and not trying to remember what I did while drunk the night before never gets old. I get so much more done without the huge time suck of drinking and recovering from drinking. I don't overspend like I used to. I really listen to my friends now and I remember what they say. I stopped hooking up with awful men while drunk and met a wonderful guy who doesn't drink much – he probably wouldn't have looked twice at me in my previous state. We had a baby last year and my son will never see me drunk like I used to see my mum drunk. I'll be the same mummy to him at night as I am in the morning. The best thing is probably that, and being proud of myself every day that I did this even though it was hard. Stopping drinking is the best thing I've ever done for myself. Being sober is great for your self-esteem!

Jane, 35

"

I used to drink alcohol too regularly for my own liking. Being a single parent meant it was only me who would finish a bottle, so even if I just fancied a glass of wine one evening, I'd end up drinking a big, fat glass for the next two evenings, too. And then it would be the weekend so I'd likely buy another bottle. The smaller bottles, with the individual glass portions, seemed such poor economy, so I'd happily glug through the standard size so as not to sell myself short. Ironic, really, considering that is exactly what I was doing on so many other levels! I have tried cutting alcohol out altogether but am not sure I really want to. Cutting back drastically instead has been life-changing enough. Waking up with a clear head has meant my coffee cravings aren't nearly so bad, either. I have noticed how much more stable my blood sugar seems to be and how much more attractive proper food is. Less alcohol = less caffeine = less blood-sugar highs and lows = less stress = stability = happiness.

Chloe, 55

"

"

I have stopped drinking for 70 days, which has been incredible. I've lost 7.5 kg (17 lb), I have been more conscious of my being, saved a lot of money and, in general, I'm just looking and feeling better. I used to get really bad anxiety for about three days after drinking and was barely able to move, to be honest – it got so bad for me that I just had to stop drinking. It's honestly the best thing I've done and all my friends around me have supported me. Some have followed suit with drinking less after hearing about the benefits.

Beth, 32

"

Having been alcohol-free now for 18 months, I've taken on two main activities. I work full-time, so this simply hadn't been possible before, when I was drinking. Firstly, I am learning Russian. I'd always had an interest in this but not the energy to pursue it. Having a little more financial freedom has enabled me to not think twice about enrolling in weekly lessons.

Secondly – and this really is a phenomenal change – my fitness has improved through running. I now regularly run up to 5 km (3 miles). From a baseline of zero for decades, now I'm 63 and very happy with this. I've lost weight (8 kg, or 17 lb, in a year) and I have been inspired to meditate each day.

I shall continue to be alcohol-free as I know there is a lot more to come.

Max, 63

"

My dad died in February 2018 and my world became a very dark place. He was my best mate and pub buddy. I have autoimmune issues and was very sick and very stressed, so I gave up alcohol to give myself the best chance of getting better physically – and also not to sink further into the abyss I was in. Dad had always maintained that drinking was a slippery slope and to be enjoyed as a treat; after he died, those words stayed with me and I really understood what he meant.

The reaction I get since quitting booze flummoxes me, though! It's something people cannot get their heads around... they either think you've got a problem or you're incredibly dull – neither applies to me. My outlook has improved since not drinking. I used to suffer crippling anxiety that was exacerbated by alcohol. Now I sleep better, I'm motivated, and my skin is clearer. It would've been easy to drown my sorrows, but I'm so glad I didn't. I want to remember my grief and all of my memories of my dad.

Maria, 42

"

"

Giving up alcohol has been the best decision I've ever made and my greatest achievement. I used alcohol to self-medicate and numb emotions I didn't know how to deal with, and to ease my anxiety (in the short-term), which only made things worse in the long-term. I have lost 12 kg (28 lb) with very little effort and feel a lot healthier. Living every day free of hangovers and blackouts has been life-changing. My mind is clearer and calmer, and I am the most at peace I've ever been. Getting sober has helped me to focus on my mental health; meditation and journaling have become integral parts of my daily routine. I have saved over £5,000 (US $6,600) and achieved some major life goals. I now have direction in my life and am beginning to really like the person I am becoming, rather than being full of self-loathing and guilt due to drinking too much. My self-esteem and self-respect have increased tenfold. My relationships have improved and I have more time to spend doing the things that make me genuinely happy.

Jenny, 34

"

"

My life has changed immeasurably since I stopped drinking in 2016. The two biggest positives have been a reduction in anxiety and being more present for my children. I was a social drinker (by that I mean, any excuse to crack open the wine), but, after having my children, alcohol caused me to suffer from crippling anxiety. I was wracked with guilt and self-loathing, my moods were all over the place, I was often teary and tetchy and felt like a terrible mother, not truly present for my kids. Almost immediately after stopping, I found my anxiety problems melted away – OK, I still have my moments, but nothing like how it was. With the more stable emotions came patience and a sense of fun, and now I have so much more time to listen to, and laugh with, my children. I occasionally still miss drinking. I miss the camaraderie of a night out, the feeling of 'taking the edge off' after a busy day, but, trust me, no glass of wine or delicious cocktail is worth jeopardizing what I have now.

Suzanne, 49

"

"

The worst thing about alcohol for me was the anxiety and panic that came after many drinking days. This stopped after a few days of quitting and has never returned. Looking back at my bloated body, rosacea-covered cheeks and lack of fitness, I realize now that I was under the spell of drinking and couldn't break the cycle. Now, as a middle-distance runner, with a clear complexion and fitness goals getting broader all the time, this shows a marked change.

I suppose the most important change, though, was giving up the belief that alcohol gave me my identity. I used to think that it was responsible for me being the life and soul of a party, the person who led the charge at the pub with the boys, the wine connoisseur at dinner with my wife... and the many other roles I convinced myself of.

After a sustained lay-off, however, I realize that was bull. I was beholden to something that limited me, and once I was free of those shackles, I wouldn't choose to put them back on.

Peter, 34

"

Booze-Free Beverages

The number of people drinking alcohol is at its lowest level since 2005, with the UK non-alcoholic drinks market having grown by 15 per cent from 2016 to 2018. More and more, consumers are keen to cut back on booze – but this doesn't mean they don't want a drink. Instead of one laced with alcohol, they want one that's alcohol-free. The choices used to be limited, but now the options are almost bottomless. A market has been created for alcohol-free drinks – and not just traditional drinks with the alcohol removed. Yes, there is alcohol-free wine, alcohol-free beer and alcohol-free gin/vodka/rum, but there are also new, innovative distilled spirits that don't try to mimic an alcoholic counterpart. They mix new flavours to offer new drinking experiences. Indeed, there's more choice than ever for those wanting to stay sober while still raising a glass. And there's a plethora of other drinks out there that won't leave you reaching for an aspirin. How about a tasty tea? An ingenious infusion? Or a palatable pressé? Ladies and gentlemen, it's time to rethink your drink.

Non-Alcoholic Spirits

The market for non-alcoholic spirits is booming. Distillers have looked at this huge drinks trend and decided to get in on the alcohol-free action. Some have created spirits that are completely original, with no intention of imitating traditional spirits such as vodka, gin and rum. Others take the core of these well-known spirits and stay as true to the original as possible in terms of taste, just minus the alcohol. Their goal is that their spirit can fit into any cocktail recipe without the need to alter the ingredients or the flavour. Gin seems to be the leader in the sheer number of brands out there, but there are many other spirits making their mark in the world of teetotal tipples.

Non-Alcoholic Wine

According to British supermarket Waitrose, sales of zero-alcohol wines rose by 64 per cent between 2017 and 2018. And in 2017, the annual global earnings from the non-alcoholic wine and beer market were a whopping $16 billion (£12 billion). That's a lot of the red, white and pink stuff. Many non-alcoholic wines are now available, with a lot of supermarkets producing their own-brand labels. It's important, however, to manage your expectations when it comes to non-alcoholic wine: it tends to lack the complexity you'll encounter in the real deal. Having said that, there are still some delicious bottles on offer that are sure to tickle your taste buds.

Non-Alcoholic Beer

From 2016 to 2018, the non-alcoholic beer market in the UK grew by about a fifth, and in just 12 months sales of high-strength beers fell by 12 per cent. It's not just bars, restaurants and supermarkets adjusting their stock: in 2018, the Great British Beer Festival offered a non-alcoholic beer (Braxzz Porter) for the first time. Consumers are increasingly health-conscious (studies have shown that non-alcoholic beers often contain antioxidants and increased vitamin B6, both of which help to prevent heart conditions) and the beer industry is all too aware of this. Many of the big breweries have jumped on the booze-free bandwagon and now produce their own non-alcoholic beers in order to satisfy those who still want a brewski, but one that won't damage their health.

Mocktails

Mocktails – non-alcoholic drinks containing a mixture of fruit juices or other soft drinks – are a great alternative to cocktails. Responding to their rise in popularity, many restaurants and bars now have a dedicated mocktail menu from which you can select your liquor-free libation. If they don't, you could always ask for a "virgin" version of a cocktail – the same ingredients will go in, just minus the alcohol. One of the advantages of mocktails (other than the lack of hangover, of course) is the price – they are cheaper than their boozy counterparts. While mocktails are marvellous to drink when you're out and about, you can also mix up your own at home. There are countless recipes, mixes and garnishes you can try out, but the following pages feature a few to wet your whistle.

Go-Go Mojito

*This combination of mint and
lime is fantastically fresh.*

INGREDIENTS (MAKES 1)

1½ tsp sugar
Mint leaves (small handful)
Juice of 1½ limes
Crushed ice
Sparkling water

METHOD

Use a pestle and mortar (or the end of a wooden spoon in the bottom of a sturdy glass) to muddle the sugar and mint. Add the lime juice to the mint mix in the glass you want to drink out of. Add crushed ice and top up with sparkling water.

Watermelon Wonder

Cool, refreshing and oh-so delicious. Great to make for a booze-free evening in with friends.

INGREDIENTS (MAKES 4)

1 seedless watermelon
120 ml (4 fl. oz) lime juice
4 tsp sugar syrup
Sparkling water

METHOD

Cut the watermelon into chunks and blitz in a blender until you have about 950 ml (32 fl. oz) of puree. Mix in the lime juice and sugar syrup. Pour into 4 glasses and top up with chilled sparkling water.

Virgin Moscow Mule

The lime gives this refreshing mule a nice kick. No vodka necessary.

INGREDIENTS (MAKES 1)

120 ml (4 fl oz.) ginger beer
30 ml (1 fl oz) lime juice
Crushed ice
Sparkling water
Sugar syrup (optional)
Slice of lime

METHOD

Pour the ginger beer and lime juice into a glass filled with crushed ice, stirring well. Top up with sparkling water until the balance of flavours is to your liking (you can also add a dash of sugar syrup if you like). Stir and garnish with a slice of lime.

SMOOTHIES

Get a hit of all things healthy with a delicious smoothie. Many of the ones already bottled contain added sugar, so why not whizz one up for yourself so you know exactly what you're putting in your body? Here are some recipes for inspiration.

Emerald Smoothie

Go green, go lean, go clean.

INGREDIENTS (MAKES 2)

225 g (8 oz) baby spinach
1 banana (peeled)
265 ml (9 fl. oz) apple juice
Juice of 1 lime

METHOD

Place all the ingredients into a blender and whizz up until smooth.

Banana and Raspberry Smoothie

This tropical smoothie is one of the most refreshing combinations you could ask for. If you want to make it really exotic, try adding coconut milk or desiccated coconut.

INGREDIENTS (MAKES 1)

2 bananas (peeled)
240 ml (8 fl. oz) pineapple juice
120 ml (4 fl. oz) natural yogurt
175 g (6 oz) raspberries
4 ice cubes

METHOD

Place all the ingredients into a blender and blitz until smooth.

Kiwi and Melon Smoothie

Zingy and sweet, super-healthy and refreshing.

INGREDIENTS (MAKES 1)

½ honeydew melon
1 kiwi fruit
1 apple
2 tsp honey
4 ice cubes

METHOD

Peel and slice the melon and kiwi fruit. Peel and core the apple, then cut it into small chunks. Place all the ingredients into a blender and blitz until smooth.

Mango, Strawberry and Banana Smoothie

A dreamy medley of flavours.

INGREDIENTS (MAKES 1)

5 strawberries
100 g (3½ oz) mango flesh
1 banana
200 ml (7 fl. oz) apple juice

METHOD

Wash and hull the strawberries. Chop the mango flesh. Peel and roughly chop the banana. Place all the ingredients into a blender and blitz until smooth.

Tea

While your garden-variety breakfast tea is a wonderful brew, it's certainly just the beginning of the story when it comes to this fine beverage. There are many varieties of tea – black tea, green tea, oolong tea, white tea, Pu-erh tea, flavoured tea, jasmine tea, chai tea, herbal tea, fruit tea, flower tea, leaf tea – all with distinctive tastes, aromas and qualities. Different teas have different benefits. Here are but a few:

- **Green tea** offers an energy boost and reduces your risk of cancer (because of its antioxidants).
- **Hawthorn tea** contains fibre and aids digestion.
- **Chamomile tea** has a calming effect.
- **Cinnamon tea** increases brain function and focus (by elevating levels of sodium benzoate) and boosts the immune system.
- **Lemongrass tea** is great for the health of your skin and hair.
- **Oolong tea** is good for your heart, brain, bones and teeth.
- **Mint tea** is a remedy for gastrointestinal issues.

Coffee

The number of coffee shops in the UK has doubled in the past decade, which amounts to one for every 3,000 people. Within them, you'll probably know that baristas are whipping up cappuccinos, flat whites, espressos, lattes, and so on. But what about the types of coffee that perhaps you haven't heard of? The weird and wonderful blends that may have even the most sophisticated coffee aficionado scratching his man-bunned head?

- **Guillermo –** Two shots of hot espresso poured over slices of lime, sometimes served on ice.
- **Breve –** An espresso served with half milk and half cream.
- **Caffè gommosa –** An espresso poured over a marshmallow.
- **Café bombon –** An espresso made with sweetened condensed milk.
- **Espressino –** A mix of espresso, steamed milk and cocoa powder.
- **Eiskaffee –** A German drink made with iced coffee and vanilla ice cream.

Water

The health benefits of water are vast. When we are dehydrated, our bodies are left lagging, flagging and sagging – and gasping for the good stuff. But what if you find water a bit... boring? Jazz it up! You can buy a host of flavoured waters these days, but often these have a high sugar content (many contain around half of your daily recommended sugar intake – yikes!). The solution? Mix your own – just add whatever fruits, vegetables, herbs and spices you fancy in a jug of water, then pop in the fridge to allow the tastes to merge. These flavourful combinations will encourage guzzling aplenty:

- Peach, lemon and thyme
- Strawberry and basil
- Lemon and cucumber
- Blackberry and sage
- Watermelon and rosemary
- Pineapple, mint and ginger
- Orange and vanilla
- Tomato, celery and black pepper
- Raspberry, strawberry and blueberry
- Orange and fennel
- Lemon and lavender
- Raspberry and lime

Infusions

If chopping up fruits, vegetables, herbs and spices to add to your water sounds like too much effort, you could always buy an infusion kit that you pop into cold water and – hey presto! – water with a twist. Some tea companies have branched out to create these packs and make different blends for that all-important yum factor. Which of these would make your mouth water?

- Raspberry and cranberry
- Orange and peach
- Passionfruit and mango
- Mint, lemon and cucumber
- Watermelon, strawberry and mint
- Blueberry, apple and blackcurrant
- Coconut, pineapple and green tea
- Lemon, orange and ginger

Bottled Bevvies

Want a soft drink that isn't one of the big-name brands? You're in luck! There are tons of delicious pressés, cordials and tonics now on the market that will satisfy your desire for a tasty teetotal tipple. And it's not just "posh lemonade" or "fancy cola" that's on offer – there are countless flavour combinations that really will create a fizzing party in your mouth. How about a cool cucumber and mint? A fruity apple and plum? A floral elderflower and rose? Or an exotic yuzu tonic water? The options are seemingly endless but, whatever you choose, your tongue is sure to be tantalized and your thirst delightfully quenched. Have fun finding your new favourite drink.

THE ONLY
PERSON YOU
ARE DESTINED
TO BECOME IS
THE PERSON YOU
DECIDE TO BE.

RALPH WALDO EMERSON

Conclusion

So, you've reached the end of this book. Hopefully you'll have taken away some advice on how to either cut back your alcohol consumption or how to make alcohol vamoose from your life entirely. Having read about drinking's drawbacks and how much you could gain from adapting (or severing) your relationship with booze, perhaps you'll be inspired to try new things. Training for a marathon? Going for that promotion? Or simply walking with a spring in your step on a Sunday? With less booze in your system, you'll be able to reclaim your weekends, restore your brain, remodel your body, recover your mental health, redeem yourself for any bad behaviour and refresh your zest.

Life isn't a dress rehearsal; you only get one shot at it. So make sure you don't ruin it with shots (or beer, or wine, or cocktails). Whatever steps you now take, make sure that you're good to yourself. If you're struggling, seek help – either from a professional or friends and family. Best of luck on your journey toward a brighter, less fuzzy future.

Further Resources

You'll find the names of a few organizations that could help you reach sobriety on page 68, and some recommendations of books relating to cutting back your drinking on page 71. Here are some online resources that you may find useful:

Club Soda: www.joinclubsoda.co.uk
Hello Sunday Morning:
    www.hellosundaymorning.org
Drink Aware: www.drinkaware.co.uk
Drink Wise Age Well: www.drinkwiseagewell.org.uk
Rethinking Drinking (National Institute on Alcohol Abuse and Alcoholism):
    www.rethinkingdrinking.niaaa.nih.gov
Hip Sobriety: www.hipsobriety.com
The Sober School: www.thesoberschool.com
A Hangover Free Life: www.ahangoverfreelife.com
The Fix: www.thefix.com
Unpickled: www.unpickledblog.com

If you're interested in finding out more about our books, find us on Facebook at **Summersdale Publishers** and follow us on Twitter at **@Summersdale**.

www.summersdale.com